I Didn't Know It Was Trauma

A Survivor's Guide to CPTSD, Suicidal Spirals, Emotional Chaos, and the Language That Finally Made Sense

Copyright Page

© 2025 Carolyn Tamm
All rights reserved.

No part of this book may be reproduced, stored in a retrieval system, or transmitted in any form or by any means—electronic, mechanical, photocopying, recording, or otherwise—without the prior written permission of the author, except for brief quotations used in reviews or scholarly work.

This book is a work of lived experience. While every effort has been made to ensure accuracy, it is not intended as a substitute for professional mental health support. The author shares personal insights and tools developed through survival, not clinical training.

Names and identifying details may have been changed to protect privacy. Any resemblance to actual persons, living or deceased, is purely coincidental unless explicitly stated.

ISBN: 978-0-473-75916-2

Printed in New Zealand
First Edition: August 2025

Dedication

For the girl they didn't see—
who felt herself dying,
screamed into silence,
and kept breathing anyway.

You were never broken. You were becoming.

And for every survivor who was invisible,
even while dying—
and for those who didn't make it—
this is your breath, your rhythm, your rising.

Wellington, 2025

—Carolyn

Opening Note

This isn't a clinical guide. It's a lived one.

I didn't write this because I have all the answers. I wrote it because I couldn't find any that made sense when I needed them most.

PTSD isn't just flashbacks and panic attacks—it's forgetting how to be a person. It's waking up in survival mode and wondering if you'll ever feel safe in your own skin again.

This book was born out of frustration—at the silence, the coldness, the way trauma gets explained like a textbook instead of a war zone. I wanted something that spoke human, not diagnostic.

If you're here, you're probably tired of being misunderstood. Me too.

This guide is for the ones who were handed trauma and told to "cope."
For the ones who googled symptoms at 3 a.m. and found

nothing that sounded like their life.

For the ones who thought they were broken beyond repair.

You're not.

This isn't polished. It's messy, raw, and sometimes dark. But it's honest. And sometimes, honesty is the only thing that keeps us breathing.

Skip around. Dog-ear the pages. Rage at the margins. This is yours.

Inside, you'll find:

- Real talk about symptoms, triggers, and what PTSD actually feels like

- Coping tools that don't require a therapist or a trust fund

- Stories—mine and maybe yours—that remind you you're not alone

- Permission to feel, to rest, to be messy, to survive however you need to

If something doesn't resonate, toss it.

If something hits hard, underline it twice.

Healing isn't linear—and neither is this book.

You're not doing it wrong.

You're doing it.

About the Author

Carolyn writes from the wreckage—where trauma isn't romantic, and survival isn't a metaphor. Her work speaks to those who've lived through the kind of pain that doesn't show up in textbooks: the invisible wounds, the forced smiles, the nights that felt like war zones. She doesn't write to inspire. She writes to tell the truth.

She knows what it means to rebuild from ruin, to reclaim softness after being hardened by necessity. Her words are a hand extended to anyone who's ever asked,
"Why do I keep feeling like this?"
"What the fuck is wrong with me?"

This book is a reckoning. It speaks to the excruciating wait times, the absence of help, the unbearable silence surrounding trauma. The pain she writes of has been unspeakable, unimaginable, and unseen—dismissed by systems that should have offered care.

The lack of acknowledgment has been decapitating and unnecessary. This should never happen—but it has, does, and will. We must learn to recognize trauma as injury: what it looks like, sounds like, feels like, tastes like, smells like, and breathes like.

We are not derelict beings to be tossed into the "loony section." That is a disgusting, inhumane, and utterly inaccurate portrayal of what we are truly experiencing.

Carolyn stands in defiance of that narrative. She offers this book as a voice for her people—for those who have been forgotten, silenced, misrepresented, and discarded. The ones left to manage their injuries alone—no bandages, no crutches, no visible proof.

If trauma were a broken leg, we'd be rushed to hospital, given time to rest, and treated with care. But when the injury is emotional, neurological, or invisible, we're expected to carry on. To explain ourselves. To prove our pain.

We are not given casts or slings. We are handed silence. We are told to "cope" while limping through life with wounds no one sees. And when we collapse, we're blamed for not being stronger.

This book isn't just mine—it's yours.

It's a map made from survival, not theory.

If you've lived through trauma and didn't have the words for it, this is for you.

Let it be a beginning.

Let it be a reckoning.

Let it feel like home.

Introduction – Why This Book Exists, and Who It's For

I wish someone had told me that surviving violence doesn't end when the bruises fade—because psychological violence *is* violence, and it can be even more devastating. It doesn't leave marks you can point to, but it rewires your brain, erodes your sense of self, and lingers in silence long after the chaos is gone.

PTSD isn't just flashbacks. It's forgetting why you walked into a room. It's rage that feels alien, shame that won't loosen its grip, and a nervous system stuck in survival mode long after the danger is gone.

I wish someone had told me that growing up with a violent, alcoholic parent and a narcissistic, emotionally absent one wasn't just "a rough childhood." It was trauma. And trauma doesn't politely stay in the past—it rewires everything. It taught me that love was conditional, safety was a myth, and my needs were a burden. That legacy didn't disappear when I became an adult. It became CPTSD. It became failure to thrive. It became the invisible war I fought every day—and still do.

This book is for the ones who've been called too sensitive, too intense, too dramatic, too needy, too high-maintenance, too hard to love.
You're not too much.
You're someone whose brain learned to survive in extreme conditions—and now it's trying to unlearn what it never should've had to know.

You don't need to be "normal." You need truth. You need tools. You need space to fall apart and rebuild without apology.

Trauma doesn't wait for the right moment. It hijacks memory, identity, and even your sense of time. And when you're in crisis, you don't need a lecture—you need something that speaks your language.

Why it matters:

- Because too many people are walking around with invisible injuries and no map, spending a lot of time wanting to die.
- Because the system keeps failing—but we keep surviving.

- Because you deserve something that sees you.

- And because healing isn't just possible—it's revolutionary.

Glossary

Trauma 101: What They Never Told Us
For the ones who never got the glossary.

Before we begin the deeper chapters, let's name what we're talking about. Because trauma doesn't always come with a diagnosis. Sometimes it just comes with silence, confusion, and a body that won't stop screaming.

This section is for anyone who's ever asked:
"Is it really trauma if no one believed me?"
"Is it PTSD if I never went to war?"
"Is it abuse if they said they loved me?"

Let's break it down.

💥 What Is PTSD?

Post-Traumatic Stress Disorder (PTSD) is a psychological response to experiencing or witnessing a terrifying event. It's often associated with combat veterans, but it can affect anyone who's lived through trauma.

Common symptoms include:

- Flashbacks or intrusive memories
- Nightmares
- Hypervigilance (always on edge)
- Avoidance of reminders
- Emotional numbness or detachment
- Irritability or sudden anger

PTSD says: "Something happened, and I haven't been able to leave it behind."

🧩 What Is CPTSD?

Complex PTSD (CPTSD) develops from prolonged, repeated trauma—especially in situations where escape feels impossible. It's common in survivors of childhood abuse, domestic violence, captivity, or systemic oppression.

In addition to PTSD symptoms, CPTSD often includes:

- Deep emotional dysregulation
- Chronic shame and guilt

- Difficulty trusting others

- A fragmented sense of self

- Persistent feelings of worthlessness

- Relationship struggles rooted in fear or control

CPTSD says: "It didn't just happen once. It happened over and over. And it changed who I am."

🏠 What Is Domestic Violence?

Domestic violence isn't just physical. It's a pattern of behavior used to gain power and control over another person in an intimate or familial relationship.

It can include:

- Physical harm

- Emotional manipulation

- Financial control

- Sexual coercion

- Isolation from friends or support

- Gaslighting (making you doubt your reality)

Domestic violence says: "I love you, but I'll hurt you if you try to leave."

🔖 Why This Matters

You don't need a diagnosis to deserve healing.

You don't need bruises to prove you were hurt.

You don't need permission to reclaim your story.

This book isn't just about definitions.

It's about naming what was unnamed,

feeling what was unfelt,

and becoming what was buried.

Table of Contents

Dedication i

Opening Note ii

About the Author v

Introduction — Why This Book Exists, and Who It's For viii

Glossary xi

Chapter 1: Where the Noise Began 1

Chapter 2: Why Didn't Anyone Tell Me? 7

Chapter 3: Unravelling in Public 11

Chapter 4: Self-Taught Survival — When the System Fails You 17

Chapter 5: Learning to Want Again 26

Chapter 6: Let's Talk Medication 31

Epilogue Companion 43

Acknowledgments 45

Books That Helped Me Stay Alive 47

Resources & Support Directory 50

Chapter 1: Where the Noise Began

They say, "Home is where the heart is."
I used to believe that—back when bedtime meant lullabies, not landmines.
But that didn't last.

Home became where the alarm bells started.
Where love came wrapped in shouting matches, slammed doors, and the kind of silence that felt like punishment.
Where bedtime felt less like rest and more like preparation—for battle, for blame, for whatever version of him or her would walk through the door.

For some of us, "home" wasn't safety—it was instruction.
We learned how to shrink.
How to disappear.
How to predict the storm before it broke.

I remember the sound of his shoes on the floorboards.
The way my stomach would drop before he even spoke.

I Didn't Know It Was Trauma

But it wasn't just the footsteps—it was the tone.
A microscopic shift in his voice, maybe half a syllable, maybe less.
I could detect it before anyone else.
I wonder if it was even audible to others.

The moment I heard it, my body would freeze.
My brain would panic.
I'd start flicking through every possible person-pleasing scenario I could enact—fast.
If I could adapt quickly enough, maybe I could soften the blow.
Maybe I could redirect the rage.
Maybe I could disappear just right.

I fucking hated it.
I hated myself.
I hated him and her.
And I hated living because of the hate.

No one told me that domestic violence rewires a child's brain.
No one explained that trauma—especially when it starts young—reshapes everything:
Attachment.
Identity.
Even how you walk into a room.

It doesn't ask for permission before it follows you into adulthood.
It just does.

I didn't look like the expected survivor.
Where I come from, violence is often racialized—framed as someone else's burden.
In New Zealand, it's easier for people to imagine trauma wrapped in the world of Once Were Warriors than to imagine a white European girl growing up with the same dread.

But trauma doesn't care about stereotypes.
My home was chaos dressed in silence.
My trauma didn't 'look right.'
So for years, I assumed it couldn't be trauma.

By adulthood, everything seemed polished.
I could function.
I had skills.
I was even considered gifted.

But inside?
It was chaos in silk pajamas.
Memory glitches.
Deep depression.

Always wanting to die but not understanding why
Big memory gaps.
Stress spirals.
Emotional skin worn paper-thin.

I didn't understand why I reacted like I did.
I just thought I was defective.
I wasn't.
I was traumatised.

🧠 How the Brain Remembers Danger

- The amygdala—your fear detector—becomes hypervigilant when shaped by early trauma.

- The prefrontal cortex—your logic and planning center—gets overwhelmed and foggy.

- Your nervous system doesn't know you're safe—because back then, you weren't.

You didn't become "weak."
You became wired for alertness.
Healing doesn't erase—it rewires.

My home trained me to expect rage, silence, guilt—then repeat.
It taught me to read micro-expressions like secret code, anticipate threats, and apologize for things I hadn't done.

That training didn't vanish when I moved out.
It got quieter.
Harder to name.
And deeply confusing to explain to people who've never lived like that.

This chapter isn't here to blame.
It's here to name.

If your home wasn't safe—if you carry childhood trauma into every adult interaction—
then your CPTSD didn't 'just happen.'
It was taught.
By repetition.
By intensity.
By the sheer unpredictability of love laced with fear.

That's not your fault.
But it is your story.
And naming it is step one.

So if you're reading this and your body still flinches at raised voices, or sounds
if you still rehearse conversations before you speak,
if you still feel like you're too much and not enough at the same time—
I see you.

You survived something that tried to erase you.
And now you're here. Naming it.
That's not small. That's sacred.

I don't want to die, and I don't want you to die either.

Chapter 2: Why Didn't Anyone Tell Me?

The Trauma of Misdiagnosis and the Double Whammy of Being Female

I bounced from admission to discharge like a poorly thrown boomerang.

Each stop handed me pills, diagnoses, maybe a 15-minute check-in.

No one said, "Hey, all this might be because you were surviving trauma for years. Your brain adapted. Your nervous system rewired. You're not broken—you've been at war."

Instead, I got told I was difficult. Disobedient. Dramatic.
One clinician said I needed to change my diet. Another implied I just needed to try harder to be "normal."
Holy fuck. The trauma of being misdiagnosed—of having your survival responses treated like character flaws—is its own kind of violence.

And if you're female? It's a double whammy.
You're told your emotions are hormonal.
Your rage is PMS.
Your exhaustion is "just menopause."
Your trauma gets buried under stereotypes about being too sensitive, too moody, too much.
Even the medical system treats female pain like a mystery—or a nuisance.

No one connects the dots between trauma and chronic, undiagnosable pain.
The migraines. The gut issues. The joint aches.
You're told it's stress, or aging, or nothing at all.
But your body remembers what your mind had to forget.

They don't tell you that CPTSD isn't just trauma—it's trauma that went on too long, with too little help, and rewired the way you feel, think, and even remember.

Instead, they toss around labels like confetti—borderline, bipolar, anxiety, depression—and expect you to stitch together an identity from scraps.
You hear terms like BPD, GAD, MDD, and wonder if any of them actually explain what's happening inside you.

But when someone finally says the word *trauma*—and explains what it does to a human being—it's like someone turned the light on in a room you didn't even know you were locked in.

🧠 What No One Told Me About CPTSD

Complex PTSD = PTSD, plus long-term emotional neglect, abuse, or instability

It often includes:

- Emotional dysregulation 😡😟🙂

- Negative self-image or guilt 😞

- Relationship struggles (trust, safety, attachment) 🤝

- Dissociation or memory gaps 🧠

- Chronic suicidality or numbness 🚫 💔

- Feeling like you're "faking it" or being dramatic 🎭

- Hormonal shifts that amplify trauma symptoms 🩸🔥

- Chronic, undiagnosable pain that no one takes seriously 🧍⚡

This stuff doesn't show up in neat checklists.

It spills out in panic attacks during small talk, deep fatigue that feels like betrayal, or the sense you're "too much" even when you're silent.

🔹 Reflection Prompt

Have you ever been told your trauma was something else—bad behavior, poor choices, or a personality flaw?

Have you ever felt dismissed because you were female, hormonal, aging, or "too emotional"?

Have you lived with pain that no one could explain, and no one seemed to believe?

Chapter 3: Unravelling in Public

What Crisis Looks Like When Trauma Is Invisible

One night, the breakdown shattered whatever fragile scaffolding I'd built to stay upright.
I was taken away in the back of a police car—not because I'd committed a crime, but because even the emergency systems didn't know what to do with someone unravelling from old pain.

I'd just been stood down from my job.
Not because I was triggered—but because I took a call where the caller named one of my family members as their abuser.
That moment cracked something open.
Not just in me—but in the system.
And instead of support, I was removed.
My employer decided I was unfit for the role.
Not because I was unstable.
But because the truth was too close to home.

I was dropped at A&E like a package no one wanted to sign for.
I waited 13 hours.
And when I was finally seen, the psychiatrist looked at me and said I needed to "learn to manage my emotions."

It felt like being handed a parachute after hitting the ground.

What I wish they'd said instead:
"Of course you're overwhelmed. Your nervous system has been trying to protect you from terror for years. You're not broken—you're exhausted."

I used to think I was just "too sensitive." That I was broken, dramatic, unstable.
But what I was experiencing wasn't weakness—it was emotional dysregulation.
It didn't come with a warning label. It came in floods: panic, shutdown, spiraling thoughts, shame.
And because no one explained what it was, I blamed myself for every reaction.
So let's name it.
Here's what emotional dysregulation actually looks like—and what you can do when it hits.

🔥 Emotional Dysregulation: What It Is, What It Feels Like, What You Can Do

🧠 What's Actually Happening

Emotional dysregulation isn't drama. It's your nervous system going into overdrive because it doesn't feel safe.
For someone with CPTSD, the brain's threat detection system is hyperactive. That means even small triggers—tone of voice, a memory, a smell—can send your system into fight, flight, freeze, or fawn.

Your body floods with stress hormones. Your thinking brain goes offline. Your survival brain takes over.
You're not broken. You're reacting exactly how someone would if they'd lived through chaos.

⚡ What It Looks Like in Real Life

- Crying suddenly and not knowing why
- Feeling numb and overwhelmed at the same time
- Snapping at someone, then feeling ashamed
- Shutting down mid-conversation

- Feeling like you're drowning in your own thoughts
- Wanting to disappear, run, scream—or all three
- Feeling like you're "too much" or "not enough"
- Struggling to explain what's happening while it's happening

🔖 What You Can Do in the Moment

- **Name it.** Say: "This is emotional dysregulation. My system is overloaded."
- **Don't chase the thoughts.** They're loud, but they're not facts.
- **Get low and slow.** Sit down. Drop your shoulders. Breathe into your belly.
- **Touch something real.** Cold glass. Textured fabric. Your own wrist.
- **Avoid decisions.** Don't text, quit, or confront.
- **Say one true thing.** "I'm safe right now." or "This will pass."

- **Let it move through.** Cry. Shake. Write. Breathe.

- **Rest afterward.** You just ran an emotional marathon.

💬 Reminder

You're not unstable. You're not manipulative. You're not weak. Your nervous system has been pushed past its limit too many times.
This isn't a character flaw—it's trauma. And it can be rewired

🧠 What Crisis Can Look Like (When Trauma Is Misunderstood)

- Panic without a clear trigger

- Emotional flooding that feels like drowning

- Inability to speak or explain what's happening

- Treated like a threat instead of someone in pain

- Hurting yourself

- Wanting to die but not wanting to die at the same time

- Disappearing

- Trying to end your life more than once—not for attention, but because the pain felt unbearable

🕯 Reflection Prompt

Have you ever reached out for help and been met with judgment, dismissal, or punishment?

Have you ever been silenced—not for what you did, but for what you knew?

Chapter 4: Self-Taught Survival — When the System Fails You

Eventually, I stopped waiting to be understood by a system that wasn't built for people like me.
I kept showing up—raw, hurting, hopeful—and kept getting handed breathing exercises by professionals who never once said the word *trauma*.

Trying to heal without naming trauma is like repainting cracked walls while the foundation crumbles.
So I stopped waiting. I started learning.

I became my own researcher.
I asked uncomfortable questions.
I explored the language of trauma like my survival depended on it—because it did.

"The biggest turning point? Finding a therapist who understood trauma—not just as a diagnosis, but as a lived experience."

📌 If This Sounds Like You...

You might relate if:

- You second-guess your emotions, wondering if you're "too much."

- You've bounced between professionals who never mention trauma.

- Relationships leave you feeling unsafe or exhausted—even when nothing's "wrong."

- You've asked, *"Why can't I just be normal?"* more times than you can count.

- You've survived things that weren't seen, weren't named, and left you carrying the weight in silence.

You're not dramatic. You're not defective.
You're a trauma survivor—and that changes how your brain, body, and emotions show up in the world.

🧠 Section: The Emotional Circuit Board

CPTSD often shows up as emotional dysregulation.
One of its most terrifying expressions? Suicidal ideation.
Not always a desire to die—sometimes just a desperate plea to stop feeling what feels unbearable.

Mental health systems often treat suicidal episodes like isolated crises.
But for trauma survivors, they're chronic symptoms of unresolved pain.

"Repeated suicide attempts don't mean you're manipulative. They mean your pain kept overflowing—and no one told you that was something trauma survivors often face."

💡 Metaphor: The Overloaded Circuit Board

Imagine your emotional system as a circuit board.

- Every wire = a relationship
- Every fuse = a boundary
- Every connection = a past experience

In a typical system, emotions rise and fall. Stress gets discharged.
But in someone with CPTSD? That board runs at maximum voltage 24/7.

- Childhood trauma frays the wires
- Domestic violence melts the insulation
- Repeated stress jams the control panel

Then a surge hits—a conflict, a memory, even a loud noise. The board shorts out. Panic. Numbness. Suicidal spiraling.

"Most clinicians inspect the appliance. Not the board. They hand you breathing techniques while the system is fried. CPTSD repair starts at the wiring—not with judging the sparks."

🚨 Common Pitfall: "Does Suicidal Thinking Mean I'm Dangerous?"

No. It means you're in pain.
Your brain is trying to escape what feels intolerable—and hasn't found a safe release valve yet.
CPTSD isn't a character defect. It's an injury to the system.
That shift in understanding? It changes everything.

🖊️ Section: It's Not Drama — It's Damage

For years, I carried shame not just for my feelings—but for having them loudly.

Every time I cried too hard, panicked too fast, froze mid-conversation—I was branded "too sensitive," "unstable," "attention-seeking."

I started believing it.

What I now know?

Those weren't character flaws. They were trauma responses. And no one saw that.

🧠 Misunderstanding CPTSD: How Survivors Get Misread

Mislabel	What's Really Happening
"You're overreacting"	Your threat detection system is hyperactive. It's protecting you.
"You're emotionally manipulative"	You learned survival tactics in unsafe relationships. That's not the same thing.

"You're always making things about you"	Trauma distorts perception—your brain scans for safety cues 24/7.
"You have no resilience"	You survived years of chaos. You're exhausted, not weak.
"You're too dramatic"	Your feelings are big—but they come from real, invisible wounds.

"CPTSD doesn't show up like a headline—it leaks into behavior, tone, reaction speed. It's subtle until it's not. And if no one understands the wiring underneath, you end up blamed for what's simply survival."

🧘 Section: Emotional Regulation — Let's Bust the Myths

Let's be clear: trauma isn't cured by calm breathing and a bullet journal.

If your nervous system is wired for hypervigilance, emotional regulation becomes a battle—not a hack.

Being told to "just control yourself" after decades of dysregulation?

It's like handing someone a map for a country they've never lived in.

🪄 Common Myths About Emotional Regulation

- **Myth 1**: You should be able to regulate your feelings by now.
  → Trauma disrupts development. Healing takes time—not judgment.

- **Myth 2**: You just want attention.
  → Expressing distress isn't manipulation—it's communication.

- **Myth 3**: You're too sensitive.
  → Your nervous system was shaped by chaos. You feel everything.

- **Myth 4**: Medication is failure.
  → Meds can be scaffolding. You're not less real for using them.

🧠 Mini Insight: Respect Starts With Recognition

When people dismiss your pain, they're not just misunderstanding you—they're erasing the invisible.
CPTSD isn't a personality defect. It's a set of adaptations forged in survival.

If you've ever been told you're "too much" for feeling what others can't see—this chapter is here to unwrite that story.

🛠 Section: So What Does Emotional Regulation Look Like?

Emotional regulation isn't about silencing your feelings. It's about making space for them—without burning down your nervous system in the process.

For someone with CPTSD, that starts with recognizing when you've reached capacity.

🧭 Trauma-Informed Regulation Isn't About Control—It's About Relief

What You Were Told	What Actually Helps
"Stay calm."	Learn your triggers and get curious—not judgmental.
"Just breathe."	Breathwork helps—but only when the body feels safe.
"Don't let it get to you."	Use grounding techniques to pull yourself back.
"Focus on the positive."	Validate your pain first. Positivity works after safety.
"Stop being reactive."	Track your emotional cycles—notice patterns, not blame.

🧰 Mini Tools That Actually Work (When You're Ready)

- **5-4-3-2-1 Method**: Name 5 things you see, 4 you can touch, 3 you hear, 2 you smell, 1 you taste.

- **Name It to Tame It**: Say what you're feeling out loud or in writing.

- **Safe-Place Visualization**: Anchor to a comforting space—real or imagined.

- **Body Scanning**: Check in from toes to head. Notice tension and ease.

- **Co-Regulation**: Sit with someone safe. Even silence can stabilize your system.

"Regulation means building enough trust with yourself to pause, to pivot, to ask: 'What do I need right now?' Every moment you show up instead of shut down? That's healing."

Chapter 5: Learning to Want Again

Reclaiming Desire, Creativity, and Aliveness

I didn't know I was allowed to want.
Not just safety.
Not just quiet.
But colour. Movement. Touch.
The kind of wanting that makes you reach.

For years, I called numbness peace.
I thought healing meant disappearing.
But it was just the absence of threat.
Not the presence of life.

Wanting felt dangerous.
Too close to needing.
Too close to being disappointed.
Too close to being seen.

But slowly, I began to notice.

The way light hit the water.

The way my body leaned toward music.

The way I craved connection—not just comfort.

I started small.

A favourite pen.

A walk with no destination.

A meal I didn't rush through.

Then bigger.

A business that reflects my truth.

A book that names what others won't.

A life that includes pleasure, not just survival.

Wanting is not selfish.

It's sacred.

It's how we remember we're still here.

Still human.

Still capable of joy.

🧭 Wanting Inventory: A Gentle Reconnection

Reader Note:

If you've been taught that wanting is dangerous, selfish, or shameful—this is for you.

You don't have to act on these wants.
You just have to name them.

Step 1: The Basics

Start with the small, sensory things.

- I want to wear…
- I want to eat…
- I want to listen to…
- I want to touch or be touched by…

Step 2: The Emotional Wants

Move into the relational and internal.

- I want to feel…
- I want to be seen as…
- I want to connect with…
- I want to forgive or be forgiven for…

Step 3: The Bold Wants

Let yourself name the things that feel too big, too tender, too "unrealistic."

- I want to create...

- I want to change...

- I want to experience...

- I want to become...

Step 4: The Truth

Circle one want that feels most alive.

Ask:

- What's one small way I could honour this today?

- What's one lie I've believed about wanting this?

- What's one truth I'm ready to hold instead?

The Anatomy of Impact

You don't need to be okay right now.

You don't need to make sense of it all.

But you deserve to understand what's happening to you.

Injury—physical, emotional, spiritual—isn't just an event. It's a rupture.

It tears through your life, your identity, your relationships, your sense of safety.

Most of us spiral not because we're weak—but because no one taught us how to read the map of trauma.

This chapter is that map.

Say out loud: "*I am here. I am safe enough. I am allowed to feel.*"
These aren't fixes. They're footholds.
They help you stay connected to the present while your mind processes the past.

Chapter 6: Let's Talk Medication

Lifelines, Not Cures

Medication isn't a fix.
It's a flotation device.

When you're drowning in symptoms, memories, or emotional chaos, medication can keep your head above water long enough to breathe, to think, to heal. It doesn't solve the storm. It gives you a chance to survive it.

For some people, taking medication feels like rescue.
For others, it feels like surrender.
And for many, it's both.

No two people respond the same way.
Some feel stabilized.
Some feel sedated.
Some feel betrayed by their own brain chemistry.
Some feel like they've finally come home to themselves.

There is no universal experience.
There is no shame in needing support.
There is no prize for suffering without help.

🌀 The Drowning Metaphor

Imagine you're in deep water.
You're exhausted. You're flailing. You're sinking.

Medication isn't the shore.
It's the life ring.
It doesn't erase the trauma.
It gives you a chance to stay afloat while you do the work.

What Medication Can (and Can't) Do

It can:

- Regulate mood and anxiety
- Reduce intrusive thoughts
- Stabilize sleep and energy
- Create space between reaction and response

It can't:

- Heal trauma on its own
- Replace connection, therapy, or self-understanding
- Guarantee the same results for everyone

My Reality: No Straight Lines

For 11 years, I was on just 25mg of Seroquel.

A tiny dose.

And it was enough.

It gave me a baseline—a soft place to land when everything else felt jagged.

Then a major life event hit.

Hard.

And I went down again.

Fast.

I'm still coming out of that one.

Still rebuilding.

Still learning what this version of me needs.

There is no linear process in healing.

No predictable arc.

Things can change in the blink of an eye—and that's not failure. That's reality.

🪄 Medication Myths: Taking It or Not

Let's name the lies. These myths have done real harm.

💊 Myths About Taking Medication

- **"If you need meds, you're weak."**
  No. You're surviving. You're adapting. You're using tools available to you.

- **"Medication is a crutch."**
  Crutches help people walk when they're injured. That's not weakness—it's wisdom.

- **"You'll be on it forever."**
  Maybe. Maybe not. Medication plans evolve. What matters is what works *now*.

- **"It changes who you are."**
  It might change how you *feel*, how you *cope*, how you *function*. But your core self? Still yours.

- **"Real healing doesn't need meds."**
  Real healing needs safety, support, and stability. Medication can be part of that.

🚫 Myths About Not Taking Medication

- **"If you refuse meds, you're in denial."**
  Not necessarily. Some people find other paths—therapy, movement, nutrition, community. That's valid.

- **"You're making it harder for yourself."**
  Only *you* know what's sustainable. Choosing not to medicate isn't self-sabotage—it's autonomy.

- **"You must not be suffering enough."**
  Pain isn't a competition. Some people endure silently. Others speak loudly. All deserve respect.

- **"You're anti-science."**
  You can believe in science *and* choose what's right for your body. Informed choice is not rejection.

- **"You'll regret it."**
  Maybe. Maybe not. Regret is part of life. So is learning, adjusting, and trying again.

🧠 Informed, Not Afraid

Whether it's pharmaceutical or natural, medication deserves informed consent.
Not blind trust. Not shame. Not pressure.

Ask questions.
Track your responses.
Advocate for your needs.
You're not weak for needing help.
You're wise for seeking support.

There's no shame in trying.
There's no shame in stopping.
There's no shame in saying, "This isn't working for me."

But please—be careful.

There are entire industries built on desperation.
Miracle healing camps.
Seven-step cures.
"Trauma detox" programs.
People promising transformation if you just surrender, invest, believe.

I'm not saying don't explore.
I'm saying: explore with your eyes open.

I say this as someone who went down the rabbit hole.
Who chased answers in places that offered relief but not safety.
Who trusted people who spoke in light but moved in shadow.
Who spent money, time, and hope on things that couldn't hold the weight of real pain.

You deserve support that respects your complexity.
You deserve healing that honours your pace.
You deserve to ask, "Is this helping me—or is it just making me feel temporarily rescued?"

🔖 Questions You Could Ask.

- What's your experience working with trauma survivors?
- How do you define healing—and who gets to decide when it's happening?
- What happens if I disagree with your approach?
- Do you believe in emotional safety, or just emotional breakthroughs?
- What's your refund policy if I feel unsafe or misled?

- Are you licensed, certified, or accountable to any ethical body?

- Do you welcome questions—or do you call them resistance?

- Can I take time to decide, or is urgency part of your model?

- What do you do when someone says, "This isn't working for me"?

Stay cautious.

🜂 Reflection Prompt

- What beliefs have I inherited about medication?

- Have I ever felt ashamed for needing it—or for refusing it?

- What does "support" look like for me right now?

🌿 Personal Note

I used to think needing meds meant I'd failed.
Now I know: they're part of my survival toolkit.
They don't define me.

They support me.
And that's enough.

⚕️ Talking to Your Doctor About Medication

A Survivor's Guide to Being Heard

You don't need to have it all figured out before you speak.
You don't need to sound "clinical" or "composed."
You just need to show up with your truth.

Here's how to make that conversation safer, clearer, and more useful—for *you*.

🛠️ Before the Appointment

1. Write down what's happening.

- What symptoms are hardest right now?
- What's changed recently?
- What's helped in the past (meds, sleep, routines)?
  Even a few bullet points can help you stay focused when emotions rise.

2. Bring your history.

- Mention past medications, doses, and side effects.
- Share what worked—and what didn't.
- Include trauma if it's relevant, but only as much as you're ready to disclose.

3. Know your boundaries.

- You don't have to agree to anything on the spot.
- You can say, "I need time to think," or "Can we revisit this next time?"

🗣 During the Appointment

1. Lead with honesty, not perfection.

You can say:

- "I'm not sure what I need, but I'm struggling."
- "I've been on Seroquel 25mg for years—it helped. But something shifted."
- "I'm scared of meds, but I'm also scared of drowning."

2. Ask direct questions.

- "What are the side effects?"
- "How long before I feel a difference?"
- "What's the plan if this doesn't work?"

3. Advocate for your pace.

- "Can we start low and go slow?"
- "I want to monitor how this affects my sleep/mood."
- "I need to feel like I have control over this process."

🧭 After the Appointment

1. Take notes.
Write down what was discussed, what was prescribed, and any follow-up steps.

2. Track your response.
Keep a simple log of how you feel—emotionally, physically, mentally.
This helps you adjust your plan and speak clearly next time.

3. Debrief emotionally.

Talking about meds can stir up grief, fear, or shame.

Give yourself space to feel it.

You're not broken. You're navigating.

🜁 Reminder

You are allowed to ask for help.

You are allowed to question help.

You are allowed to change your mind.

Medication is a tool.

You are the expert on *you*.

Epilogue Companion

This poem was written in 2007, during a time when my inner child first began to stir. It waited patiently for me to return. Now, she leads the way.

Awakening Child

by Carolyn

Release my great stone—it is heavy in here.
I need to taste laughter; we are craving fresh air.
My soul made of tears, I beg me no more.
My search—is it lost? We can't find the door.

Are we punished or tainted? I don't understand.
A fight lives within me to remain with this land.
She has sampled the light and delighted my mind—
A child, like stillborn, holds breath it can't find.

It's bursting and thrusting with gladness through veins,
But the devil delivers like a deep-seated stain.
Where are you, my girl with pretty blonde curls?
I feel you inside me, dancing on pearls.

Are my hands on your ears so you are not me?
It's important you listen if we want to break free.
Together we grew, but drifted apart.
Your light is still shining—I'm here in the dark.

We are counting on me to let your self in.
Awakening little child, let our journey begin.

Acknowledgments

To my dad—

You were both my tormentor and my teacher.

In the end, you chose to see. You chose to listen.

And in those final years, we found something rare: honesty, tenderness, and a love that neither of us expected.

Thank you for meeting me there.

You gave me something I never thought I'd have—a place to land, and a reason to stay.

To Andy—

Your quiet steadiness, your patience, your presence over thirty years—those things held me when nothing else could.

You were a lifeline I didn't know how to name.

And even if the words never came, your loyalty reached places in me that nothing else could.

To anyone who ever stopped to listen—without fixing, without judging—you have no idea how many times you saved my life.

Your kindness was oxygen.
Your silence was safety.
Your belief was enough.

To every reader holding this book:
I care about you.
I don't care about your race, your gender, your sexuality, your past, your pain, or your paperwork.
I care that you're here.
I care that you're still breathing.
I care that you're trying.

This book was written for you.
Not the polished version.
Not the "recovered" version.
The real you.
The messy, aching, brilliant you.

May these pages be the moment someone once gave me—
a moment of listening, without judgment.
A moment that says:
You matter. You're not alone. You're allowed to exist.

Books That Helped Me Stay Alive

Healing isn't something I did alone.
It came in fragments—through books, questions, voices that reached me when I was barely reachable.

These are the works and thinkers that helped me find language, sanity, and a way back to myself.
I share them not as prescriptions, but as possibilities.
If even one of these speaks to you, let it.
Let it be a spark.

📚 Books, Thinkers, and Teachings That Held Me

- **Byron Katie – *The Work***
  "Who would you be without the thought?" cracked open the space between reaction and reality. It gave me breath.

- **Nathaniel Branden – *The Six Pillars of Self-Esteem***
  A framework that helped me rebuild the foundation trauma tried to erase.

- **Clarissa Pinkola Estés – *Women Who Run With the Wolves* & *Warming the Stone Child***
  Myth, story, and soul-deep remembering. Her words felt like ancestral medicine.

- **Melody Beattie – *Codependent No More***
  A mirror I didn't want—but needed. Her work helped me untangle my worth from my wounds.

- **Jasmin Lee Cori – *The Emotionally Absent Mother* & *Healing from Trauma***
  She gave language to the ache I couldn't name. Her work felt like being seen.

- **Gabor Maté – *In the Realm of Hungry Ghosts* & *The Myth of Normal***
  Compassionate, unflinching truth about trauma, addiction, and the nervous system.

- **Bessel van der Kolk – *The Body Keeps the Score***
  A reminder that trauma lives in the body—and that healing must, too.

- **Dan Siegel – Attachment theory & interpersonal neurobiology**
  His work helped me understand the wiring beneath the wounds. It gave me context, not blame.

I Didn't Know It Was Trauma

Resources & Support Directory

For Survivors, Seekers, and Those Still Surfacing

You've made it through the pages.

Now here are places to turn when the noise gets loud again.

This list is not exhaustive—but it's a start.

You deserve support that listens, believes, and adapts to *you*.

🆘 Emergency & Crisis Support – New Zealand

Service	Contact	Notes
Need to Talk? – 1737	Call or text 1737	Free, 24/7 support from trained counselors
Women's Refuge	0800 REFUGE (0800 733 843)	Crisis support, safe housing, advocacy
Shine	0508 744 633	Domestic abuse helpline, safety planning
Lifeline NZ	0800 543 354 or text 4357	Confidential support for distress, suicidal thoughts
Safe to Talk	0800 044 334 or text 4334	Sexual harm helpline, anonymous and trauma-informed

🌐 Global Helplines & Survivor Networks

Service	Region	Contact	
RAINN	USA	1-800-656-HOPE	rainn.org
The Survivors Trust	UK	thesurvivorstrust.org	
Blue Knot Foundation	Australia	blueknot.org.au	
Hot Peach Pages	Global	hotpeachpages.net	

🧠 Trauma-Informed Therapy & Education

- **TherapyRoute.com** – Find trauma-informed therapists worldwide

- **NZ College of Clinical Psychologists** – nzccp.co.nz

- **ACC Sensitive Claims** – Support for survivors of sexual violence in NZ

- **The Mighty** – Survivor stories and mental health community: themighty.com

- **Blue Knot Resources** – Guides for survivors, professionals, and supporters

🗡 How to Vet Safe Support

- **Trust your gut.** If something feels off, it probably is.

- **Ask about trauma training.** Not all therapists understand CPTSD or DV.

- **You can leave.** You're allowed to walk away from any service that feels unsafe, invalidating, or coercive.

- **You don't owe full disclosure.** Share only what feels right. You are not a case file—you are a person.

www.ingramcontent.com/pod-product-compliance
Lightning Source LLC
Chambersburg PA
CBHW062043290426
44109CB00026B/2714